Inspired

7 Steps to Your Most Inspired Life

DYLAN M. MILLS

East 26th Publishing
Houston, TX

First printing edition 2019

East 26th Publishing
Houston, TX

www.east26thpublishing.com

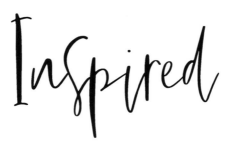

Inspired

7 Steps to Your Most Inspired Life

To my daughter, Raleigh

The girl who inspires me every single day with her kindness, stubbornness, and unique sense of fashion.
May you never lose that sparkle, sweet Rammer. Xo

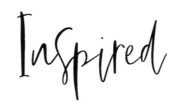

Inspired

7 Steps to Your Most Inspired Life

Introduction

INTRODUCTION

For many months, I racked my brain trying to come up with a title for this book. What do I title a book with which I intend to start a movement?

"I want this book to inspire women…"
"I want women to be Inspired to make positive changes…"
"I want women to be Inspired to lead their best lives…"

That one word *Inspired* just kept reappearing.

Have you ever looked up the definition of *Inspired*?

I needed to make sure this powerful word that kept circling my thoughts proved to be as mighty as I felt it to be.

Inspired: **Of extraordinary quality, as if arising from some external creative impulse.**

Wowza.

Anyone else get chills, or is that just me?

I'm reminded of a childlike quality when I read these words—of a mental state knowing the world is limitless; you have everything ahead of you; you can pursue any dream, no matter how outrageous. And that's exactly how it should be.

Reading those words, I want you to think —

How *Inspired* is *your* life?

When you wake up in the morning, are you jumping out of bed with your goals set, excited to kick off the day? And I don't mean like on the one day in 4th grade when you got to take a field trip to Sea World. I don't mean on Christmas morning when you want to run downstairs and see your kids' faces light up. I mean every. single. day., sister. Are you waking up every single day feeling excited and ready to chase your dreams?

Are you moving forward with an "external creative" drive? By this, I mean, is there something outside of your day-to-day bubble that is pulling you forward, helping you grow, and utilizing your most creative talents? Is there something yanking on your heartstrings and begging to be done? Do you have dreams outside of your comfort zone just waiting to be chased?

Are you living your most extraordinary life?

Are you truly utilizing this life and living it to the fullest?

Are you setting an example for those around you?

Is your life *Inspired*?

If your answer to any of these questions is "No" or "Meh...,"
then this book is for YOU.

As children, we are so quick to believe in ourselves, in our
possibilities, in the possibility of what's ahead. The question
is, at what point did we begin to lose that sense of limitless
possibility in our lives? When did we decide that "going
through the motions" and "just getting by" are okay?

When did we stop being *Inspired* by our dreams, goals, and
personal potential?

This is my most recent epiphany. An epiphany that drove me
forward to creating this book for you.

Maybe you have faced challenges and obstacles. Maybe life
has thrown you a few curveballs that have knocked you
down. Or, maybe nothing tremendous has happened at all,
but you just feel stuck in the spin cycle. And sister, that
stinks. I mean, tragedies, loss, and complacency are not
easy. But, do you know what's even harder? Being stuck.
Staying in that place for the rest of your life does not serve
you, and it does not serve those around you.

As hard as this pill is to swallow, it's the truth. Negative things
will happen again. And again. And again. And that may not
be what you want to hear, but sister, we're human. And that's
life. Simple as that. We can't prevent these things from
happening to us, but I can help you learn how to move
forward NOW.

What I want to do is help you live. Like, really live. I want to
show you how your mindset, your actions, and your outlook
can change everything. I want to help you take control of your
life and utilize these best practices going forward.

I'm not claiming to be some all-knowing, self-help guru. But what I am saying is that if we work together, we can end the cycle of ho-hum thinking and living.

Together, we can transform ourselves and those around us to be truly Inspired.

Yes—work, laundry, dishes and carpools will all still have to be done. Instead of dreading those tasks and going through them with monotonous disdain, let's complete every mediocre task with an extraordinary sense of positivity and pure, unadulterated JOY.

Let's work together on focusing outward to find a sense of power and purpose in serving others, in empowering others, in inspiring others.

And then, let's get down to it, lady! Let's figure out what it is that you dream about. What it is you fear (and perhaps society has told you) you just can't do.

Now, before we dive into the actionable steps and walk through everything you need to know to start your Inspired journey, I think it's important to take a step back in time to help you understand my personal journey.

In order to do this, I'm going to need to level with you—and as I do this, I need you to promise that when it's your turn you're going to do the same. Deal? (I fully expect that you're at least nodding your head at me while reading. And if you're not, just give it a shot... Humor me, will ya?)

Okay, so now that we've gotten that out of the way, I'm going to admit something to you that I struggled admitting to myself for many years.

My name is Dylan… and I am a recovering control freak.

Now, as I say this, I don't want you to think that I've left this part of me behind. I am still a control freak at heart. But, I have been able to implement the strategies that I am going to teach you in this book to balance out my need to control outcomes, and apply those strategies when things don't go how I planned.

In the past, my constant need for control became a massive, debilitating problem in my life. My life-long battle with anxiety has often caused me to function improperly. For me, the constant need to control outcomes, to control my future, to control *everything* has been the source of some major anxiety struggles all through my childhood and into my adult life. Like an alter-ego, my calm, cool, collected demeanor instantly morphs into my alter ego, who, for humor's sake, I like to call "Deb."

Things didn't go how I meticulously envisioned them?
Deb gets hit with a nasty sour stomach.

The restaurant didn't have the chicken fingers I wanted?
Deb is brought to tears.

Learning I had less than 3% chance of conceiving?
Sorry about it. Deb experiences the ultimate hyperventilating, life changing breakdown.

You guys, I literally used to bring Tums with me at all times because of how often I would get anxiety. Over nothing.

Finding out I might not be able to get pregnant—that was my turning point.

That was when I realized I couldn't keep living this way.

That last one was where I truly desired a change.

That last one was where my controlling, planning, anxiety-ridden-self had the hardest time grasping what to do next. When I say breakdown, you guys, I mean BREAK-DOWN. Tears, hyperventilating, researching every possible scenario in which others beat the odds. You have no idea how many chat forums and crazy stories are out there.

When my husband and I got married, we had already been together for four years, lived together, adopted a dog, and gotten through the "I can't believe he thinks that's how you load the dishwasher" phase.

We. Were. Ready.

And you know how in high school you hear all the sex-ed teachers talk about how *easy* it is to get pregnant? How basically just looking at the opposite sex has already implanted that baby, and if your cycle is like 5 minutes late it probably means you're already pregnant, and what are you going to do, how do you tell your paren—Phew, maybe that was just me?

Well it didn't happen like that for us.

And then it didn't happen the next month.

And remember that control freak I discussed earlier? Deb let her anxiety flag fly high, y'all.

"I read here that if we both eat pineapple it will help."

"I read that if we stop drinking it will help."

"A woman said her husband took vitamins and it worked."

On, and on, and on. Every month a cycle. Hope, impatience, calculating that if this were the month, then the baby would be due in... —and then crushing defeat.

Finally, we saw my doctor and he ran some tests, and was able to tell us that he knew why we weren't getting pregnant (control freak Dylan immediately perked her ears up at this). Basically, he said we wouldn't be able to get pregnant without the help of a fertility specialist.

I won't go into every moment from that time, but I think you get the idea.

B.R.E.A.K.D.O.W.N. central.

Here's something I want you to understand, though:

Breakdowns are *not* an ending.

Breakdowns are *not* your defining moment.

Breakdowns are the beginning of BREAKTHROUGHS.

Let me repeat that.

Breakdowns are the beginning of BREAKTHROUGHS.

Now, sure there are scenarios in which you want to wallow, choose to wallow, and stay wallowing longer than necessary. But, sister, these types of moments are the perfect opportunities for a positive change.

This is the perfect moment for you to allow INSPIRATION to take hold.

During that time of breakdowns and disappointment, I felt a calling to just take some kind of steps in a positive direction. That control freak needed something to control when so much else was going out of her control.

So, I did what any twenty-something would do.

I got on Instagram.

And guess what?

I took a plunge into something terrifying.

I started an online business focused on my own health & wellness and got totally out of my comfort zone. Rather than wallow and continue to wreak havoc on my life with my futile attempts to control, I turned my breakdown into a breakthrough.

During that time, we continued our attempts at getting pregnant, but at least I had something else to focus all of my energy on. The business I created became my baby.

And after months of tests, appointments, and long drives to the specialist's office, we got pregnant with our first miracle baby during a month that we had to "take off" from our next scheduled round of fertility treatments.

That month off—the month off that I almost couldn't cope with—ended up being the month my beautiful girl was conceived. And you know what? At 14 weeks postpartum, we found out we were expecting our second miracle baby, without the help of any treatments.

And guess what?

Because I didn't get pregnant when we were trying originally, I started an online business.

Because I started this online business, I was able to cut back hours at my day job when my son was born.

And now I am able to retire from teaching at 28 years old and stay home with both of my children. Working from home, writing in the early hours of the morning, and soaking in all of the work-from-home mom perks.

Breakdown turned breakthrough.

If I hadn't gone through that breakdown, I would never have had the courage to break through.

We would still be living paycheck to paycheck, paying my entire salary in daycare bills, not able to be regulars at our Friday morning music class. Those are things I will never take for granted.

I tell this story not to give you a full play-by-play of my fertility journey, but to tell you this: Your breakdown is something to embrace, to soak in, and to break through.

That's exactly what I want to dive into during the rest of this book. How to take your breakdown moments—no matter how crushing—and turn them into your own breakthroughs.

How to take that control freak, Deb, give her a glass of red wine and tell her Taylor Swift style that she needs to "calm down."

And then take on the challenge of living every single day, Inspired.

In the next four weeks, I want you to be selfish and unselfish. I want you to take time for exercise, for self-care, for reflection, and for dreaming. I also want you to take time to serve, to spread joy, and to be the change. Your change.

I want you to learn how to take control of your life by letting go of what doesn't serve you.

I want to teach you how to alter your mindset when things don't go as planned.

I want to show you how to fill up your cup, so you can pour into others.

I want to help you schedule joyful activities like an appointment you can't miss.

I want to encourage you to take big scary steps toward your dreams.

I want to motivate you to create your healthiest, happiest version of you.

In the next four weeks, I want to start your movement toward healthy and empowered living.

In the next four weeks, I want you to be INSPIRED.

Let's do this.

XOXO,
Dylan

Step One

Step One

LET GO OF CONTROL

In order to take control of your life, you're going to first need to let go of the idea that you need to control everything.

Now, I know it may seem counterproductive to hear me say "We're going to take control of your life!" And then five minutes later hear the complete opposite. Let me explain how these two ideas work together.

When my sister and I were very young, my parents divorced. Let me immediately point out that, as much as I love both versions of the movie, we were NOT the kids from *Parent Trap* crafting ways to get our parents back together. For Emily and I that was just the way it always was.

They have both been remarried for a long time and have given us so many siblings that my heart wants to burst with love. I literally can't imagine anything different. However, I will say this: Being a child who constantly goes back and forth on weekends and holidays is not easy. Yes, it has become more of a norm in today's society and, yes, I was lucky to have so many safe homes, but it still wasn't easy.

As I've told you before, I have suffered from anxiety and "Deb attacks" since I was a child. I think part of this stemmed from a lack of control in my home life. All children have, and rightfully should have, a lack of control when it comes to their home life. Ultimately your parents should in fact be in control of keeping you healthy, safe, fed, and loved. For me, the stress came to fruition because I wanted to decide everything for myself. So, this anxiety and unnecessary stress was purely my own doing, not the result of any kind of instability in my homes.

Let me stop really quick to point out something important here. This fact that my anxiety—the panic attack, rock in my stomach, made me want to puke anxiety—was my own doing. Deb came into play here, even at a young age.

If you have never suffered from anxiety, it's easy to say, "But everything is okay," "But you're safe," "Just stop thinking about it," etc. And I promise you that I have sat there and reassured myself in the same ways. But there's just something, some inkling, some thought, some smell, some-something that brings about a sudden panic. This can manifest in all different ways, in all different people, and honestly it can feel out of body. No matter how much you reassure yourself, there's this feeling that just won't quit. Deb, or whoever your mental battle monster is that keeps prodding and bringing up your fear, your lack of control, that one possible scenario, that thing you did wrong over and over and over again. It's a vicious cycle. And for me this anxiety tended to stem up in moments in which I felt out of control.

One of my family's favorite stories to tell is when five-year-old me convinced Emily that we were going to have a Mary-Kate and Ashley style adventure, hitch a cab, and head straight to the Embassy Suites for Happy Hour popcorn and Shirley Temples. I can still remember Emily crying into her suitcase as she lifted a picture of our mom, kissed it 10000 times and placed it ever so carefully amidst the two dresses, barbies, and blankie that were already inside.

I kicked the screen out of our bedroom window, and off we went to the driveway—because, if you didn't know, the end of a quiet, residential neighborhood driveway is exactly where the best cabs are hailed. It didn't take long before my stepdad found us outside and immediately brought us in. When he inquired just how we were expecting to pay for this illusive cab and hotel stay, I quickly retrieved the paycheck I had stolen off of his dresser. Yes, you read that correctly folks. And I have yet to live that down to this day.

In other instances, I can remember having gut wrenching anxiety every Saturday night when Prairie Home Companion came on the radio, because I knew that meant a new week was coming and that anti-change Deb monster inside of me couldn't stand the uncontrollable changes ahead. Even little things like getting an invitation to a birthday party would make me instantly nervous because I wasn't sure whose house I would be at that weekend. Therefore, playing out the entire weekend in my head was totally out of my control.

I had my first actual Panic Attack (I mean—gulping for air, breath after breath and feeling like you're suffocating) when I was eight. I vividly remember being at my dad's house, in the wood paneled room that Emily and I shared, having a dream that I was watching myself sleep from the perspective of a fly (Odd, but not even close to the craziest dream I've ever had). As the fly descended and landed on my chest, I immediately woke up and felt like the air had gotten knocked out of me. I legitimately thought I might die. I was gulping, gasping, trying to get air and felt like nothing was working. It was a nightmare. When I finally got myself out of bed, I woke my dad. I remember sitting with him on the front porch in the pitch black of night, for who knows how long. We just sat there on the wooden swing out front and waited for my panic attack to subside. That was my first, but not my last.

I went through so much of my childhood, teens, and early adulthood assuming that this was normal. I also assumed that this was how my life would be... forever. Any situation that did not go exactly how I meticulously envisioned it going, would bring about anxiety. This was not something I frequently spoke about out loud and, honestly, it wasn't until just recently that I was able to combat it.

I share all of this because maybe you have experienced panic attacks, lack of control, or maybe you were also an avid Mary Kate and Ashley fan and, like me, failed to realize how irresponsible they were in many of their movies.

So, let's talk about how to LET GO in order to move forward. Here's the idea that I want you to manifest:

Control the controllable. Make the most of the rest.

Let's break down what this idea means. When situations in life happen that are not in your control, are not how you envisioned, or not what you wanted, you can either give in to defeat and crippling anxiety...OR, you can try to make the most out of the situation. Now, I will tell you right now, this does not mean that any and all anxiety is instantly eliminated. Instead, what I am wanting to help you do is control how you react when anxiety rears its head. You cannot control the situation, but you *can* control how you react to it. Even when anxiety bubbles up, you can take a deep breath, make a short list of what's right in that moment, and figure out what you *can* control in the situation. Then let go of the rest.

When I graduated college, I incorrectly assumed that I would be a hot commodity and land my first teaching gig after my first interview. Ha. Ha. Ha. That was not the case you guys. On one hand, I was amazed at the number of interviews I was able to land, and yet completely discouraged by the number of job offers I received in return (a whopping ZERO).

Deb haunted me.

What if I don't get a job?

What if I'm just not cut out for this?

Then one day I decided to stop moping and get outside of my bubble. I sent out emails to multiple schools in surrounding counties. I got a call immediately for an interview at a school about 55 minutes away from my house. I was going from an internship at an A+ rated school to a teaching job at an F rated school. (For those who don't know, these ratings are determined by test scores. Generally, the more funding, parental involvement, and teacher retention the school has, the better rating the school will get. But that's a topic for another day.) So, this school was way out of my comfort zone, but I got the job! And honestly, it was the best thing that could have ever happened to me.

From that one uncontrollable instance, I was able to begin my teaching career with more compassion, behavior management training, and appreciation than I would have gotten anywhere else. Yes, there were difficulties. Yes, it was heartbreaking to hear my students say they didn't eat anything all weekend. Yes, I broke up a fight between two first graders on my second day in the classroom. And, yes, my classroom was infested with roaches. But I grew.

My mom has this quote that she shares with me frequently throughout my life, and in this instance it became a mantra. "Bloom where you are planted." In this particular instance, I wasn't planted in the high-end school I envisioned, but you know what? I bloomed. I made friends, I made a difference, I learned more about myself and the education system than I could have learned anywhere else. And THAT is where letting go of your need to control can take you.

Where are *you* planted right now?

Are you in a job, home, or situation of any kind that isn't ideal? Or maybe your headspace and anxiety are taking residence in your mind and keeping you stuck? Well, guess what, sister?

Nothing is going to change if you don't change.

If you don't let go of the things that don't serve you; if you don't relinquish control of the uncontrollable—you will never bloom.

When I was in my first classroom, I had to learn to control the controllable and let go of the rest.

The classroom was dirty. There wasn't a real bulletin board and there was no carpet for my kids to sit on. Great. I cleaned it, I created my own bulletin boards, and I put stickers on the faded tiles to give my students assigned places to sit. I couldn't control what happened to those students when they left school at 4 pm. But I could control their environment when they were with me. I could support them, teach them, love them, and give them my all while I was there.

I have learned to control the controllable and let go of the rest. If I can't change something, I am only hindering myself by harping on that thing. Why waste my time if it is totally out of my control?

If you have children, you can relate to the fact that we absolutely cannot control them. I can make the most delicious meal, slave over a hot oven (or microwave) and present a perfectly plated meal to my daughter, and guess what? I've learned there is a 95% chance that she will decide that today she's actually not into those egg muffins she loved yesterday. So, instead, the dog eats her carefully distributed scraps and I'm left feeling defeated. Sound familiar to you?

Except, here's the kicker: I have learned to let go of that defeat. Sure, it pops in my head, but one deep breath and a moment of reflection is all it takes to reset and make the most of the situation. I can control what I feed her, but I can't control what she does. This is a lesson that has been implemented many times raising babies. I can't control how my toddler reacts to situations, but I can control how I react. I can't control when my newborn son wakes up in the middle of the night, but I can control my own sleepy emotions about it and embrace every snuggly moment in his reclining chair.

What is something you are having difficulty letting go of?

What's a situation that you hold on to and just can't seem to move away from?

Or, maybe there's nothing massive. Maybe you just can't seem to get out of your "stuck" place? Maybe you just don't know what to do to move forward with life in general?

On page 6 of your Toolbook, take two minutes and simply record your answers to these questions based on whatever comes to your mind first.

What is out of your control?

What is holding you back?

There is zero judgement attached to any of these things as you record them. I just want you to identify these things so that you can let go and move forward. Now, once you have identified your uncontrollables, let's identify out how to apply this lesson to your everyday.

I cannot control the traffic, so does it serve me to get emotionally attached to the fact that I'm running late and these cars are all on the road with me? I mean, how dare all these people also try to get to work? Don't they know I'm running late to music class? Sister, the answer is no. And as much as we'd all love to *Bruce Almighty*-style wave our finger and get those other commuters out of our way, we can't. And that's okay. Look at the situation you're in and decide what part of it you can control. Most of the time, the answer is going to be: You can control how *you* react to the situation.

Instead of getting anxious and angry, you can turn on a podcast that you love and listen while you have the extra time in your car. You can jam to your favorite playlist and have a mini dance party while you sit in traffic. Or, you can leave 10 minutes earlier tomorrow and try to avoid it altogether.

Can you see what I'm getting at here? In every uncontrollable, WE are the controllable.

So, all my fellow control freaks out there—there's good news. While we are in fact going to practice letting go of control, you are still going to be able to take the wheel like the backseat driver that you are.

Here's what I want you to practice: When a situation arises today that is out of your control, and anxiety starts to creep in, I want you to stop, take a deep breath, and decide how this moment is going to serve you. Can you change the thing that is happening? If you can, great! Make a change. If you can't, great. Let's decide what you *can* change. Whether it takes a change of your own plans, a change of clothes, or a change of your mindset, do it.

What I want you to do now, before we move forward, is to go back to your Toolbook and find those uncontrollables you wrote about. I want you to go to every single one of them and write down something you *can* control in those situations.

Here are examples from my own journaling:

I can't control my daughter's big emotions, BUT I can control the way I react to them.

I can't control when my son will wake up, BUT I can control the level of enthusiasm and love I exude when he does wake.

I can't control other people's opinions of me, BUT I can control what I listen to and how I let it affect me.

I can't control the line at Starbucks, BUT I can control the positive conversations I have while I stand in line.

How does that feel? Personally, letting go of control and embracing the fact that I am not an omnipotent being that is in charge of everything and everyone...is a HUGE relief.

Taking hold of what I can control and letting go of the rest is the most freeing thing I've ever done.

Step Two

Step Two

MASTER YOUR MINDSET

Your mindset determines everything.

Let me repeat.

Your mindset determines everything.

How crazy is that?

How POWERFUL must our mindsets be to determine how *everything* else will turn out?

Your mindset determines the way you handle every single situation in your life.

I want to set a little scene for you here. A few years ago, before I started practicing all of the steps that I'm explaining to you here, there was a morning I slept past my alarm and did not get my usual morning "me" time. My kids were the ones who woke me up, they were both in disastrous moods. It was raining outside, so it took extra-long to commute to my teaching job. Oh yeah, and my husband was out of town, so I was wrangling kiddos solo, running to work on empty. Phew, it was a doozy. And guess how that affected the rest of my day? I think you can imagine. I was in a horrible mood, and no matter what happened, I handled it with the same negativity with which I started the day.

This may sound like a typical morning for you, or maybe you don't relate at all because you're always in a good mood—in which case, you're the unicorn we've all been looking for. It's so normal to get into a bad mood. Sister, every single day your mind goes through cycles of up and down. Some days may have more ups than downs. Some days you may wake up on top of the world, and then all of a sudden your coffee spills all over the cute top you've been dying to wear, you get stuck in traffic on the way to work, and the Starbucks line is way too long for you to even think about going through the drive-thru. Total downer. Totally normal. But...

What if you could retrain your brain to handle these outside circumstances with poise and positivity?

What if you could retrain your brains to take in these situations, evaluate them for what they are, and attach ZERO negativity towards the rest of your day?

Well, you CAN.

When you are able to detach the situation from yourself.

Looking at these situations objectively and deciding to remove negative energy will help transform how you handle these situations from now on.

On that day when I was running late and didn't get my "me" time in the morning, I chose to ruin my day. I didn't enjoy the moments around me, I didn't take time to smell the roses and embrace what was good. I didn't even control the controllable things. I just let that negativity spread like lice in a kindergarten classroom and I did nothing to stop it.

What should I have done?

I should have stepped back and assessed what was going on with me. I should have reset my mindset, recalculated my day, and embraced the fact that even though so much was going wrong, everything was alright.

I have found that in these moments, the best thing I can do for myself is take a moment of Thanks. This can be done on paper, in your mind, or even quickly typed out on your phone. A moment of Thanks is taking one minute to think of as many GOOD things as you can. Even though everything may be going wrong, what *are* you grateful for in this day, or in this moment? What can you give Thanks for? What blessings can you embrace in this moment, in this day, in this life? Taking a moment of Thanks can reset your entire mindset and quickly turn it from negative to positive. It can take your mindset from a place of despair to a place of hope. At the very least, recalling all the good in your life can calm you down and level you out.

I remember after having my daughter, I immediately assumed I would bounce back, feel amazing, and be able to function on this "little sleep" that people always talked about. I mean, hello, I went to college. I went to sleep at 3 a.m. and woke up ready to function at 7 a.m. It's like I had been training my entire life. Ha. Ha. That was *not* the case. Breast feeding, postpartum hair loss, a baby with massive gas issues, and very little sleep for mom and dad made it nearly impossible for me to function as normal. I set really high expectations for myself and when I couldn't meet those (unrealistic) expectations, I was devastated.

Let me give you another example.

As I got ready to go take our newborn pictures, I did a kind of crazy tribal dance trying to pull on my pre-pregnancy "stretchy" jeans. HA. And let me say, getting them on was the easy part. Seeing that extra fluff hanging over was heart-wrenching. Mind gut number one.

Then, while trying to do my hair and makeup, I found that my normally thin hair was even thinner. One may even say that my newborn daughter had more luscious locks than me. The hair line I was experiencing was that of a middle-aged man about to go through a midlife crisis. *What was happening to me!?* Mind gut number two.

Then, the end all, be all. The cherry on top of the cake.

I had on a shirt that was just flowy enough to hide the mom bulge…and my daughter spit up all over it. Out of an entire closet of clothes, this was "the only one I could wear." I was angry, hurt, tired, and just exhausted from everything going wrong. Mind officially gutted.

Y'all, my mindset was a wreck.

This beautiful, joyous day that was supposed to capture a glowing moment in our lives was completely ruined.

Now we all know it was, in fact, not ruined. But that's not what I thought.

After that last bomb, I immediately began combing through my brain for a list of scenarios in which I could postpone the pictures—yeah that will work. I'll just give it another 6 weeks until I'm clear for workouts, load up on ALL of the B vitamins, perhaps even get some of those clip-in extension things I keep seeing everywhere—yeah, obviously our only solution.

My husband was not on board. Our sweet photographer (and friend) was ready for us, and I needed to get it together.

You guys, my mindset almost ruined that special day for me and for my entire family. And you know what? Every time I look at those pictures, all of those feelings come rushing back.

During a moment that I should have been grateful and full of joy, I was self-conscious, upset, and devastated by the morning's events. Talk about disappointing. And it was not the fault of my muffin top or my jeans (that must have shrunk in the wash). It was not the fault of my precious hair, or my daughter's less than ideal cookie-tossing.

No, it was my fault.

I let those situations get the best of my mind.

I let my negative mindset get the best of me.

I was the one who decided how I would handle it.

Instead, I harbored every single thing that was not going my way, that was not working in line with my perfectly typed and highlighted plans for the day; instead, I decided that those outside factors would determine my day. However, I could have decided to take control of my mindset. Remember that control we talked about in Step One? This is it. Could I change all those scenarios? No. But I could change my outlook. I could have changed how I was seeing things, and focus on the good, the grace, the positive.

What I should have done was taken a moment of Thanks and embraced what was so good. This baby girl we had prayed so stinking hard for was in my arms. I had multiple outfits I could have changed into. We were getting amazingly free photos from a sweet friend. I mean, hello, the fact that we were in a home we owned with food and a roof over our heads, surrounded by love—that should have been enough. And maybe in that instance I needed to take multiple moments of Thanks. That's okay! Do what you need. Bringing yourself back to a place of love and calm within whatever storm you're battling will prevent you from ruining beautiful days of your life.

You can't decide what happens to you, but you can decide how you let it affect your mind.

Sure, you can play out a scenario, think about how you want it to go, but there are so many outside factors at play that you, in fact, do not control. Remember, we're letting go of those uncontrollables anyway! And, yes, it can be challenging to fully grasp how little control you have of situations. Here's the deal, though. While you cannot control other people, freak accidents, or your child's bodily functions, you can absolutely control your mindset by taking negative moments and twisting them into a positive. You can take moments of disappointment, embarrassment, or even anger, give Thanks, and let that re-route you to a better place.

Your state of mind is one of the most important aspects of this entire book.

Maybe right now you're already conquering your health, your job, your income, and checking all the boxes, but something is still missing. On paper, you are succeeding, but there is something internally that won't allow you to let go and appreciate it all. And if you can't be intentional, present, and joyful, that affects everything and everyone around you.

Have you ever been on an airplane and watched as they go through the "in case of emergency" instructions? What is the thing that they always tell you if those oxygen masks come swinging down? PUT YOUR OXYGEN MASK ON FIRST. You cannot serve the person next to you if you can't breathe. You cannot save your child if you are not safe.

In order to live Inspired you also need to learn how to take your everyday tasks—the ones that you possibly dread doing but know have to be done (I'm looking at you, laundry), those ones that seem to get in the way of your day—and turn them into opportunities instead of obligations. Your goal is to create a strengthened, Inspired, clear mindset that is focused, creative, and able to process anything that comes your way.

Anytime I mention mental states like this (joyful, present, intentional, clear, Inspired, etc.) people don't think of all the mundane day-to-day tasks that don't immediately sprout "JOY." And, sis, I get it. I really do. But if you cannot find joy in your day-to-day, you are wasting it.

You will never have that exact day back again. You will never have that moment with your child again. You will never have that date night again. You will never have that exact night out with friends again. If you cannot be in a positive, present mental state in these moments, then you are wasting them.

When you look back on your life and the moments that collectively make up the collage of you, what will you see? Think about the time leading up to this very moment. What are the first emotions, occasions, memories, feelings, smells, sounds, that pop up in your mind?

Take 3 minutes right now to journal on page 13 of your Toolbook. Is there a word you see used repeatedly? Is there an age, a moment, or a specific memory that reoccurs? What feelings are attached to that?

Now, thinking of these moments, I want you to give yourself pure, unadulterated grace. Even if you look at those scenarios and feel nothing put pain and remorse, you are still here. You still have this day, right now, in front of you. You get to decide from this moment on, how you want to spend your time. RIGHT NOW, sis. You get to decide HOW YOU WILL LIVE.

When hard things happen, how do you want to react?

When life sends you curve balls, how do you want to handle them at the plate? (Baseball analogy say whaaaat. My husband will be proud!)

When we were about a week out from our wedding day, it rained. And I don't just mean a little sprinkling thunderstorm, I mean Florida style monsoon rained. There was flooding all around town, including our wedding venue. This beautiful wooded area, with the perfectly envisioned accents and rustic feel I had been dreaming of...was flooded. The long dirt road that led back to the venue was undrivable, and we received a phone call explaining that we may want to look into other options. One week out, you guys.

Let me relay two different scenarios for how this was handled:

Deb—you know her, right? That control freak alter-ego, besties with your anxiety, always looking for the worst. Well, she went into full panic mode. "The wedding is ruined! How will we afford another venue? What about the table settings and everything I planned? How is this even going to work!?" Immediate anxiety, popping Tums like tic tacs. Still teaching and letting this negativity head into her classroom space. Deb was not present. Deb was worried. Deb was spending her precious teaching time in the classroom focusing on what was wrong with her venue and worrying about what would happen. Deb had a full-on breakdown amidst the fake florals lining the hallway of her local Hobby Lobby.

Dylan, on the other hand, made a list of Thanks and embraced a positive mindset. Dylan knew that even though the venue might not work out, everything would be alright. Dylan knew that, even though things were getting out of her control, where you get married is nowhere near as important as who you're with. She knew she'd be surrounded by family and friends, and it would be beautiful no matter what. Dylan was intentional in the classroom, present with her students, and used her time with them as an outlet. She focused on the positive things happening in the classroom and made moves forward after school to find other venues.

Spoiler alert. Parts of both of these are true. Luckily, our wedding venue dried up two days before the wedding with enough room to get to the rustic lodge and our outdoor ceremony. Did I change that with my worrying? Did my stress serve me in that situation? (See what I'm getting at here?)

Read through these scenarios and apply them to your life. Which mindset takes control when obstacles occur?

How can a positive mindset change your perception?

When you read about these two women, which one do you relate to most?

Which one of these is the current YOU?

Which mindset do you gravitate towards more?

Now, take out your Toolbook and complete the next activity on page 16, noting that this is NOT a time for self-criticism or negativity. We are human. There is no "wrong" answer here. There is nothing wrong with you.

Take a moment and reflect. Feel free to journal any thoughts in your Toolbook in the space provided. Can you think of moments in which your mindset has altered activities, events, or even bad news?

Either way, this is YOUR TIME, sister. Find solace and peace in knowing that moving forward, it's only going to go up from here!

This is not to say that life won't "happen."

Things will get tough. You will face many trials. But what I want to help you do is create schedules and practices that will help you process these obstacles with a clear heart and mind.

Step Three

Step Three

FOCUS ON THE INSIDE

In this next section, we are going to continue focusing INWARD.

I realize that in today's society, we are classically conditioned to believe that too much inward focus makes us selfish. We are often raised to believe that thinking of ourselves is wrong. And I will be the first to tell you, that this guilt is real. Reading through the first parts of this book, you may have already had thoughts about how much time and effort you are spending on YOU. Ever heard of "Mom Guilt?" (It's real, btw. Still waiting to hear back about "Dad Guilt" though...) But I think this is a similar concept. I think so many of us suffer from *"ME* GUILT."* What is this thing that I decided to put in italics AND all caps for you? Well it's something I think plagues a lot of people, especially women. We are taught so often that to think of ME is wrong. Doing something for ME is wrong. Chasing a goal for ME is wrong. And if we do decide to do these things, or chase those dreams, or think of ourselves and our mindset at all—that we are selfish. I'll be honest, my biggest way to justify (because, apparently, in my mind, I'm constantly on trial for every little thing I'm doing) is to say, "But I'm doing this because if I run this marathon, I will be a better mom." "I am a stay at home mom and am dropping my kids off at a home daycare because I am chasing this dream and passion that, in turn, will serve them because I'll be a better mom."

What if I'm chasing this dream purely because it's mine?

What if I'm running this marathon because I want to prove to myself that I can?

Is that so wrong? Wouldn't you applaud your daughter or son for chasing after that same thing? Wouldn't you be eternally proud of your sister or BFF for doing that same thing? Wouldn't you RAISE THE ROOF in the biggest way possible, if YOUR MOM did the same thing?

So, why is it wrong if YOU do it?

Well, guess what? It's NOT WRONG.

And I may catch some slack for that, but I will stand firmly planted right here because I truly, in the depths of my heart, believe that what you DO and what you BELIEVE have a direct impact on your life and everyone around you.

Your mindset, your outlook, your well-being, doing something that brings you joy is just as important for you as it is for other people. You with me?

Okay, so in order to take some massive action, I need you to go ahead and air all your dirty laundry. I know for a fact that as women we very quickly drive our minds to come up with limiting beliefs the second dreams pop up. Whether it's fear of judgement, fear of failure, or that wretched "me guilt," it pops up and tries to slam you down.

What are your doubts, fears, or limiting beliefs? Journal your answers on page 23 of your Toolbook

For me? It was doubt in my abilities and fear of failure or disappointing others. And my limiting belief was that I wasn't worthy of more because other people may not approve.

Say whaaaat?

I'm going to tell you one lesson that I learned very quickly when I started living without those beliefs.

You are not everyone's cup of coffee.

Want me to repeat that?

You are not everyone's cup of coffee.

You cannot add a dash of almond milk and a spritz of pumpkin spice to please everyone.

You also cannot water down your flavor and add soymilk in order to please people.

If you are an Iced Vanilla Latte with a sprinkle of cinnamon and caramel drizzle, BE THAT, sister!

Don't dilute yourself to a plain ol' cup of coffee just because you think that's what everyone wants.

Don't you dare limit your dreams and visions for YOUR LIFE based on your fear of what others may think.

As I watch my kids' personalities emerge more and more every day, their natural dispositions become clearly apparent.

My daughter is shy and determined. She has a sweet, calm, mothering disposition that just comes naturally. She has the independent spirit of her mama, with a love for the outdoors like her dad, her own creative ideas and a brilliant little mind that is all her own.

My son, on the other hand, is a ham. He is friendly, loud, and active. He is obsessed with his big sister and does everything he can to get her attention. He moves, laughs, and plays nonstop. And when it's time to sleep, he's out like a light.

These two children are their own people.

And when I look at those lights that shine through each of them, I cannot imagine ever dimming them. And when I imagine either one of them coming to me and telling me that someone else doesn't like how they are or coming to me questioning who they are because of other people, it makes me want to cry. I mean, honestly, my mama heart shatters into 10,000 tiny pieces thinking of either of my babies ever feeling like they are not enough.

And, sister, if we feel that way about our own children, then why would we ever think that way about ourselves?

If someone tells you they don't like something about you, what do you do?

Do you change to fit their expectations? Do you LIMIT yourself based on what they like?

Do you water down your cup of coffee because it's too strong for them?

The easy answer would be, "No, I would never do that," but seriously think...

Has there ever been a time in your life where you have changed, lessened, or increased something you do because of what other people think? Journal your thoughts on page 25 of your Toolbook.

When I was in middle school, I can remember very clearly some instances of this starting to occur for me. In my mind, middle school is created purely as a holding ground for the most awkward years of your life. Go ahead—get braces, acne, and play with all the Mary-Kate & Ashley eye liner you want (is that even still around?) and we'll all just do it together and look back and cringe. I was right there in the thick of it. And y'all.... I'm about to share, probably one of the MOST EMBARRASSING anecdotes of my entire life, and you know what, we're just going to laugh about it together.

When I was in seventh grade I was right there at the height of awkward preteen-ness. I wore my hair in braids every night because I wanted that highly fashion-forward "crimped" look to be rocked with my Abercrombie jean skirt and the "motor mouth" shirt I had at the time. Not TOO bad yet, right? Well, let me also mention that my naturally inclined body type has been brought forth by the male side of my family. This body type includes noodle arms and legs with any weight that might hang on for dear life, doing it right to your midsection. Along with that, I was cursed with zero backside. I mean, y'all, no chest is one thing (have that too) but the derriere is a whole different animal and something I didn't even realize I was "supposed" to care about. I was so naively unaware of any of that until one fateful day. I was in the bathroom with friends (because, as every female age 12-21 knows, you cannot go to the bathroom by yourself, duh), standing in front of some full-length mirrors and hearing someone compliment a friend of mine on her "bubble butt." "What does that mean?" I naively asked. This is the part where, in a middle school musical version of my life, girls would have broken out singing *Baby Got Back*.

I can vividly remember turning to my side and looking in the mirror and replying, "Yeah, I think I have a bubble butt too."

(Insert your very best impression of preteen snickering here)

"Dylan, you definitely don't. Your butt is like totally flat."

Y'all, the American Eagle stitching on the back of those skinny flared jeans could not have felt any tighter. So, what do you think this gal did? Take a wild guess... and even then, you're probably not going to guess right.

Have you ever heard of girls stuffing their bras?

Well, sweet, young, bubble-butt-less, middle school Dylan stuffed her pockets.

I mean, genuinely in the worst, most obvious way possible. Y'all, it makes my pulse race just thinking about it. I grabbed some of my pads—PADS, YOU GUYS—and I PUT THEM IN MY BACK POCKETS. Not just for one day, but for the rest of the school year. And no one ever mentioned it. You read that correctly, ladies. I stuffed my pockets to give the (terribly unconvincing) illusion that I, in fact, had back, baby.

And why did I do this? Something I was woefully unaware of came to light because others cared. I didn't care about what my backside looked like until I realized other people did.

Maybe you're not stuffing your pockets, but I can guarantee there's some other way that you're altering your appearance, your disposition, or your personality to fit other people's expectations.

Fast forward to high school years, when my intense craving to please other people intensified. I was carefree and also insanely insecure. I remember hearing through the teenage grape vine that someone said that they didn't like me because I was "always laughing and trying to make other people laugh, and it's just annoying." So, anytime I was around this specific person I tried to tone myself down. I took all the water I could and tried to dilute that delicious almond milk latte that I was deep down. And guess what you guys? That did not make me happy. It actually did the opposite. I was so worried about, "Was that too much?" "Did I laugh too hard?" and it sucked out my joy.

I'm going to tell you right now. A watered-down latte does not taste good.

SO, STOP WATERING YOURSELF DOWN.

What I want you to do now is think of ALL of the things that make you, YOU.

What are those elements of yourself that you can define?

What unique, identifiable characteristics do you see in yourself? Journal about it on page 25 of your Toolbook.

Now, turn that into your own personalized cup of coffee. Take a moment to visit page 26 of your Toolbook and create your perfect cup of coffee—the YOU that only you would order.

Maybe there's an aspect of yourself that you want to work on.

Maybe you are too quick tempered, maybe you worry too much, maybe you want to work on being more confident—those are up to you, and only help brighten you. If you are going to change something about yourself, it needs to be because you decided to change, not because other people want you to. There is a quick difference here if someone does ask you to change something that negatively affects those you come in contact with on a daily basis—a quick temper, a judgmental spirit.

When that happens, I want you to think: *Is my ____* (whatever quality) *bringing someone else harm?* If it is, then the decision to change needs to come from you. Then it needs to happen. It needs to happen because you know that harming others is not going to serve you or anyone else, ever.

The point is, when you decide that your cup of coffee is enough for you, then you can find inner peace.

This extends to your actions as well. The things you do or dream of doing should not be dictated by other people, but instead by your own innate desire to do them.

Want to color your hair? Awesome, do it.

Sally will probably love it because purple is her favorite color. Janice will probably hate it because she thinks purple hair is tacky. WHO CARES about either of their opinions? Are they walking around with magical purple hair? No, you are. If you like it, and you're not harming anyone else with those luscious locks of yours, then WHO CARES? ENJOY IT.

Want to run that marathon? DO IT.

Want to buy that cute jumper? DO IT.

Want to apply for that job? DO IT.

Want to write that book? DO IT.

Heck, want to sell all your things and live the van life? DO IT. More power to you. But just make sure that you are doing what you want, not what you think other people want you to do. This, sister, is where your true potential and happiness are revealed.

So now that we've talked about it, let's get real girlfriend. I want you to look deep down inside to the core of who you are. To do this, you are going to make two different lists.

As you begin working toward living your Inspired life, it's important to create a vision of what you want that life to look like. It's vital to know who you are, and what makes you tick. You defined your innate characteristics and who you are by creating your cup of coffee. To do that, let's dig into some actions that bring you joy.

On the first list (page 27 of your Toolbook), you are going to list five things that made you happy as a child.

Maybe that was playing house, going for bike rides, playing sports, playing board games, etc.

On the second list, I want you to list five things you love doing now. Five things that you want to make room for in your life. Five things that are taking up room on the back burner. Five things that you're too scared to do. Five things that make you feel Inspired.

That wasn't so hard was it?

Do you see any similarities between the two lists?

Feeling Inspired yet?

Don't worry, we will come back to these things soon enough.

Step Four

Step Four

SERVE OTHERS

Now that we have focused INWARD, it's time to change scenery and focus OUTWARD.

What do I mean by this?

In order to live your most Inspired life, you cannot have a purely self-centered focus.

It is vitally important that you take time for you. I will tell you that a million times over. But balance is also vitally important. So, in this section, I want you to figure out some simple, day-to-day ways to serve those around you. This could be anything from paying it forward in the Starbucks drive thru line, to asking the barista how her day is going, or even greeting someone else in line with a smile and a compliment.

Focusing OUTWARD means that you are helping, serving, Inspiring, and having a positive impact on others. Service and a heart for helping others is one way to bring ultimate purpose and passion to your life.

Serving others can mean big tasks like going on a mission trip, serving at your local homeless shelter, or even volunteering at a local park clean-up. Or, it can mean small daily tasks like smiling at everyone you pass on the street, bringing coffee to your coworker, showing patience and kindness to everyone you interact with during the day, or being a good listener. The craziest things happen when we are able to spread positivity and love to other people, even in ways that seem so small.

When I was in college, I worked multiple jobs to support myself while living in an apartment with friends. If I'm being honest, there were moments in which I was bitter because so many other people around me (friends, classmates, etc.) didn't have to work. They received any and all funding from their parents. However, looking back, I wouldn't change a thing because those jobs made me who I am today. They helped me learn how to stay focused, they made me humble and they helped me build compassion. As a struggling college student, I worked at a church nursery two mornings a week, did the school pickup scene every day, and also worked at a self-serve frozen yogurt store. And yet, I was still overspending and budgeting poorly. Little things that I took for granted began to weigh down on me—especially driving.

At the time, I drove a Jeep Grand Cherokee. It was my dream car, and I was obsessed with it. But it got 14 miles to the gallon. I would drive as little as possible because I couldn't afford to fill it up all the time. I learned how to judge the gas light and how long I truly had until it would run out. I learned that if there was not enough money on my debit card (Hi there, $3!) and I needed gas, I could run my card as credit, and it would let me spend it—over drafting my account but giving me gas. Y'all, these are things I would break out in cold sweats about, yet, I was too "prideful" to share with anyone.

This brings me to a particular day that I had counted up all the change I could find to fill my empty tank. I was close to tears. I was running late for work and was about to head inside to the attendant and ask him to put $2.75 in my pump so I could get a gallon of gas. Out of nowhere, a sweet elderly man at the pump on the other side of mine turned to me and said "Excuse me, hun, I don't know if you want it, but I have a full tank and still have some money left here. Would you want to fill your car up with the rest of this?" You guys, I cried. That sweet old man helped me reach the pump to my car and fill up my car with SEVEN WHOLE DOLLARS of gas. We started talking and I told him I was going to be a teacher, and he said he was helping volunteer at his church's Vacation Bible School. He invited me to join in, to which I quickly relayed how absolutely busy I was. Instead of hammering it anymore, he handed me a VBS Card with cartoon jungle characters all over it and said that if I changed my mind there was a spot for me.

I have kept that card all these years to remind me how special that moment was.

It reminds me that even though we don't know what's going on in other people's lives, we have the ability to help them— big or small. That man probably had no idea how much he helped me that day. That small act completely changed my day. It completely cheered my mood, and I decided right then and there that I wanted to be able to do that for other people as often as possible.

I challenge you to think of a time right now (maybe one already came to mind) when someone did something so kind and so unnecessarily out of their way that completely turned your day around?

I want you to be that person for someone else. Who knows what that person in front of you at the grocery store has been going through that day? Perhaps she seems rude or judgmental, when in fact she just received terrible medical news about a close family member and she's just angry and trying to process. So, if that same woman quickly cuts in front of you in line, how do you respond? With anger and disdain? Or, can you respond in that moment with kindness, gentleness, and a smile? Can you ask how her day is going? I promise it is the most rewarding thing to pay it forward and serve others, especially when they are at their worst.

Sometimes I think we assume that servitude has to stem from something massive—like donating a kidney or selling everything you own and moving to a third world country. And while those things are absolutely amazing, they may not be realistic for you right now. They may not even be the service you're called to do at all. There are so many more, small scale things that can serve people in your community. Ripples can create waves. Your simple act of smiling at a neighbor is a ripple. Imagine if that gets paid forward 10,000 times. You have a WAVE, girlfriend.

Another way to serve is through your work. Is there something that has been placed on your heart, in your soul, in the depths of your being that you just love doing?

Perhaps this calling is your form of servitude.

Love playing piano? Maybe you can volunteer at a local nursing home to share your gift and lift spirits once a month.

Are you called to work with children? Then being a teacher may be your calling, working with students every day to mold them into incredible human beings.

Maybe you're an amazing artist? Create some art that you can give away as gifts for others.

Honesty, maybe you just have a contagious smile? You can use that gift every single day to lift the spirits of those around you.

It doesn't matter how you serve, whether it's a big task or a small one. IT ALL MATTERS.

That is why I created this section of the book. I think so many times we go through books, videos, courses, and podcasts like this, finally ridding ourselves of that "me guilt," fired up after flying through chapters and episodes, convicted and ready to change our lives, and, yet, the focus on changing other people's lives as part of the equation is often missing.

You guys, this is a VITAL part of the equation. Even on your worst days—heck, ESPECIALLY on your worst days—you HAVE to make a conscious effort to focus on lifting up others.

So, with that said, let's dive into how you can implement this!

On page 35 of your Toolbook, list five things that you are good at and enjoy doing.

Now take those talents and turn them into five ways you can serve others.

Reflect. How often are you currently doing these things?

Are you leaving time to Inspire others?

Or, is there an imbalance between your inward & outward focuses?

As you move into the next parts of this book, you are going to dive deeper into your Inspired life. You will be taking these lists and ideas and creating a schedule that you will be able to implement each and every day.

So, with that, let's move on, girlfriend.

You're doing great!

Step Five

Step Five

HAPPY HOUR

Raise your hand if you love a good Happy Hour!

Cute outfit, all the chats and giggles, a nice big glass of wine, maybe even 2-4-1 right now?

Well this kind of Happy Hour is going to be a little different than your usual drinks out with the gals. (Although, girl, we can *totally* chat about this over a glass of Prosecco anytime!)

This kind of Happy Hour is a daily homework assignment.

We talked about how important it is to change your mindset. Accordingly, one thing I truly believe makes the biggest difference in your life is having time for yourself.

Scheduling a TIME just for you.

This time is to be used however you want.

Be honest. What was your immediate reaction when you just read the word "Homework?"

I can almost hear the *womp womp* of your disappointment.

But not to worry! This homework is all about you and your happiness.

Want to go for a run? Want to finish knitting that sweater? Want to just lay in a bubble bath with your favorite jams playing? GREAT, SIS. DO IT!

Is your first thought, "I don't have time to do that!"?

Yep, that used to be my way of thinking too. But, sister, this is *your* LIFE we're talking about. As we discussed earlier, you only get this one, and, honestly, if you truly want to live your most Inspired life, you have to schedule in your Happy Hour.

This is about making time for yourself and your life. This is you time. This is just for you. To bring in happiness no matter what others think. This is where your mindset centers and you reset. This is the time you're able to control. This is time just for you.

Have I said that enough already?

Now I realize some schedules allow for more flexibility when planning this out, but regardless, it's vital that you make it work however possible, girlfriend. If it means getting up an hour before your kiddos, DO IT. If it means putting aside work at night to take a little time for yourself, DO IT.

Now, maybe an hour seems totally daunting right now. I totally understand that work schedules, kid schedules, newborn life, you name it—they are all crazy and demanding. So, maybe start smaller.

Maybe start by scheduling in 15 minutes (and, girlfriend, if you can't get 15 minutes a day to yourself, then something major needs to change). 15 minutes for you to walk, rest, meditate, write, journal, run, whatever your happy hour task is that day.

When I first had my daughter, I totally neglected this time. I was so caught up in the newborn fog and lack of sleep that "me time" was no longer in existence. And guess what happened? My tank ran empty. I got to a point in which I was literally in tears, bawling my eyes out, with a precious nugget on my chest, trying to feed her, while she cried right along with me. We were a mess.

Finally, I spoke to my husband finally and said, "I just need 15 minutes." 15 minutes of silence. No crying, no one needs me. It was hard the first time because I was immediately thinking of all the things that they both probably needed me for while I was in the other room (Remember the "mom guilt" I talked about earlier?). I remember thinking that I was the worst mother in the world because I needed time away from my baby—extremely critical and self-deprecating thoughts. And then I fell asleep. When I woke up with a start, 30 minutes later, I ran out in the living room to find my husband and daughter giggling and doing tummy time together. Guess what? They were fine without me. And that unintentional 30 minutes of me time made me so much happier and more present when I was with them. From that point on, I vowed to always take some time for myself. So, I created my very own Happy Hour.

When you think of getting an entire hour to yourself, what do you imagine doing?

And laundry, dishes, and cleaning DO NOT count, you over achiever, you.

No. What do you LOVE to do, but never have time?

Need some help thinking of joyful things you can do?

Look back. Remember earlier in the book when we discussed those things that make you happy? Check out your list! We talked about our childhood happy activities and about current happy activities, and now you are going to take those and make time for them during your Happy Hour.

As I mentioned, I made a vow to myself to take my Happy Hour every day and did this as I could. And then, at 14 weeks postpartum, I found out I was pregnant with miracle baby number two. And my energy levels took a nose-dive. By the afternoon, when I was normally taking my Happy Hour time to work out, journal, etc., I was having trouble just keeping my eyes open. So, I sat down and rearranged my schedule and decided to START my day with my Happy Hour. Y'all that 30 minutes of me time, has now transformed into my alarm clock going off at 4:30 a.m. DAILY, and yours truly jumping out of bed like a jack rabbit to go sip my coffee in my office, do my devotional, journal, and plug in to something that makes me happy before the rest of my crew wakes up. It has become an absolutely vital part of my routine.

Maybe you're not a morning person. Maybe you read that and said, "Oh heck nooooo." Maybe you would rather stay up late? Great! Good for you. So, schedule in a nonnegotiable Happy Hour for yourself every evening.

I will say, if you schedule this time and find that, much like me, you end up repeatedly skipping it because life is happening (as it dares to do so often), then I challenge you to wake up earlier. Start small and work your way up to your full hour in the morning! It may seem challenging, maybe even dang near impossible. But, sister, I PROMISE you it is worth it.

Making it a part of your routine will change so much of your day and give you the time to chase after something you love. On page 43 of your Toolbook, make your list of Happy Hour activities. What can you spend that one hour doing?

Now, looking at these activities and decide which ones are realistic for you to incorporate daily. For example, maybe going to brunch with girlfriends makes the list, but it's not realistically something you can do every single day. Then schedule brunch with your girls weekly or monthly instead! Set a date and make it happen!

Doesn't that feel better already?

Well, hold onto those butterflies, sister, because we're about to dive back into the scary stuff.

It's time for....

Step Six

Step Six

THE FEAR FACTOR

I'm not going to ask you to lay in a bed of snakes or eat worms. NO. Instead, I'm going to ask you to do something much scarier. We're going to dive into those scary aspirations you hid away in the back of your dreams.

Wipe away those cobwebs and let's get scheming!

Raise your hand if you have ever heard the expression, "You can't have it all." (If you're not raising your hand right now, you better raise it high girlfriend).

Okay, how about, "You can't have your cake and eat it too."

Guaranteed you've heard at least one of those sayings, and I'm 95% sure that you've believed it, at least a little. I have lived so much of my life hearing sayings like this and assuming them to be true, without even questioning what my ALL would be.

I have told myself things like:

"You can't be a good teacher and have other dreams."
"You can't be a good friend and a good girlfriend."
"You can't be a good mom and run a successful business."

I can think of 1,000 more examples from my entire life. And now, all I can think is, "WHY NOT?!"

Why can't I be a good teacher, dreamer, friend, girlfriend, mom, and entrepreneur?

Because someone else said I can't?

Oh, no.

When I was a kid I had about 12 trillion different ideas of what career path my life would take.

Actress. No, Dentist. Actually no, Teacher. Strike that. Cast member on SNL? Eh, actually I would love to be a Lawyer...

When we were young, my mom would take out a notebook once a year and write down our answers to various questions like, "Who is your best friend?" "What's your favorite food?" and "What do you want to be when you grow up?" My sister was always spot on with either a dolphin trainer or teacher (She's currently getting her PhD in Early Childhood Education, so shout out to her). However, if you were to go through all of those years of responses, mine was different every. single. time. Perhaps the best response I ever had was in our Fifth Grade Yearbook.

Want to know what my response was?

A teacher, a lawyer, or an FBI agent.

You can get off the edge of your seat; My FBI career has yet to take off. Although, I have done some serious stalking for friends about to go on blind dates.

My mom is a teacher. I grew up around the school. I love working with children. So teaching was my obvious choice when entering college. They don't have a major specifically made for *Good Morning America* co-host, so Early Childhood Education took my attention.

My first glimpse in the realm of "you can't have it all" was while in college.

I stayed in my hometown, along with many friends from high school. I tell my husband all the time, college was basically High School 2.0 for me, including shamefully skipping classes, one of which I failed because college Dylan didn't realize there was a pop quiz during every class. When I finally showed up to one and was handed a quiz, I, being extroverted as I am, turned to the people around me and said, "PHEW, good thing I came to class today." Which was immediately met with, "Oh my gosh, you know we have quizzes after every single lecture, right?" I'm pretty sure my face turned the color of my daughter's favorite wagon (Red, if you didn't catch that).

See the problem was, if I was going to go to class, I would be missing out on time with friends who didn't have class at that time (Rock solid logic, I know).

I was also working three jobs in order to support myself in the apartment I shared with a couple other friends. I would head to my job at the self-serve yogurt shop and feel guilty because I wasn't going out that night with friends. I would want to go to a class at the gym in the morning, but I would feel guilty because that means I wouldn't be able to stay up late with my roommates or go out to whatever bar they were planning on going to that night. I would hang out with friends and feel guilty because I wasn't with my family while they watched a movie. I would hang out with my boyfriend (now husband) and feel guilty because I wasn't out with friends that night. I assumed the obvious answer was just "You can't have all of these things." I would do one thing and hear disappointment from whoever I wasn't with.

I wish I could go back in time and give that stressed out Dylan a gigantic bear hug and tell her, "It's OKAY." When we believe the adage "You can't have it all" and assume we need to choose one thing over another, our friendships, family relationships, and romantic relationships all suffer.

What I should have done, was explain to every party that I had things I wanted to do.

I should have explained how important my feelings were and set my own priorities and boundaries.

When I started teaching, I soon realized that, as much as I loved my job and being in the classroom, I also felt drawn to more. I racked my brain for what that might be. And then one day an opportunity presented itself to join an online company. This was around the same time that my husband and I were trying to get pregnant, that control freak Deb was in her element, and I had so much doubt in myself and my abilities that I was nearing a mental breakdown.

"I can't do this and teach."

"I can't work a business and take time away from my husband."

"I can't miss social gatherings in order to pursue a dream."

Well, guess what? YES. YOU. CAN.

And you should.

When I first decided that I wanted to do something outside of teaching, I was a nervous wreck. I mean, I went to college for four years to get my degree. I had finally nailed a job at my dream school. Why on earth was my heart calling for more? At this same time, my husband and I were going through fertility treatments and trying to start our family. And I was thinking about adding something else to my already full plate?

Yes, yes I was. This dream was one that was unconventional and honestly got some kickback. "You're joining one of those companies?" "What's wrong with teaching?" "Why are you posting so much on social media?" The questions came from many people that I considered close friends at the time. I began to doubt myself along with them. *Maybe they're right? Maybe I shouldn't do this? Maybe I'm not meant for more?* All the maybes, doubt, and insecurities rang through.

Y'all, my best friend at the time stopped talking to me and unfollowed me on all social media because she said she was annoyed with "that kind of stuff." RIGHT THERE. That would have been a reason to quit. But guess what? I kept going. I decided right then and there that I was going to prove all of the doubters wrong. I was going to take this and build my dream. I was going to live the life that I had always dreamed of instead of living someone else's. And honestly, I am forever and ever thankful that I did.

This calling is on your heart for a reason. This DREAM is on your heart for a reason. And just because THEY may not understand it, they should still support it. Who cares if you post ten sweaty selfies on your Instagram? Are you hurting anyone? No. Who cares if you want to leave your teaching job even though you had always dreamed of teaching? Are you hurting anyone? No. The point is, it's your dream. You don't need to limit your dreams just because others don't have the same one.

Your dreams are just as important as everyone else's. And I'm going to tell you something that may not be the most popular opinion, but it has been my truth.

If people don't understand it, or support you—if people you thought were your friends unfollow you on social media and start talking about you behind your back if you aren't able to attend a social event, then those are not your people.

My husband was skeptical of my ability to balance all of the things, and I won't say I have been perfect 100% of the time, but I've tried. I wake up to work in the early hours and, for the first three years, still went to the classroom during the day. The important thing is that we communicated about it.

If you want to have your version of "ALL," then you need to be open to communication, especially with those around you whom it may affect.

If you want to chase a big scary dream, then have that terrifying conversation and just know that your *real* people, your tribe, your support system should and will support you.

Yes, I could go back to those old feelings of guilt, but instead I've chosen PRESENCE and INTENTION as my focus. If I'm working, I'm all in. If I'm playing with my kids, I'm all there. If

I'm with my husband on date night, I'm embracing that time with him. In order to have your all, you need to let go of the idea of perfection. You also need to let go of the idea that you can't have dreams and be a mom, wife, sister, or friend. SO, let's dive into this for you.

Have you ever looked up the definition of "Fear?"

Honestly, I hadn't ever consider looking it up until working on this part of the book. So, I just whipped out my dictionary and...just kidding. You know what I just did? Laying here on my bed, completing this part of the book, I called to Alexa and asked her to define it for me. If that isn't spoiled, I don't know what is.

In all seriousness, the definition looks something like this:

Fear: An unpleasant emotion caused by the belief that someone or something is dangerous, likely to cause pain or is a threat.

Let me get real with you. That "book" that you want to write... Is it a threat? Is it dangerous? Is it out to get you or harm you? So why are you fearful of getting started?

What about that Zumba class you've been dying to teach? Unless the participants are middle-aged zombies waiting to snack on your brains, I'm pretty positive none of them are out to cause you any harm.

So why in the world do we let FEAR dictate so much of our future? Journal about this on page 49 of your Toolbook.

Why do we live in a constant state of worry about what harm, hurt, or failure might fall unto us?

When I was little, I dreamed of going on the Tower of Terror ride at Hollywood Studios in Disney World. I saw it every time we approached the park and every single time, I dreamed of being brave enough to ride. You see, I love scary movies, I love books with psychological twists and turns, and I had seen the Tower of Terror movie that Disney made, which basically sealed the deal right there (If you haven't seen it, go find it in the depths of Disney history and watch it!).

So, there came a day when I finally plucked up the courage. My siblings (who are all younger than me, I might add) were going to go as well. We waited through the hour-long twisting and turning line and found ourselves in the basement area watching earlier line-goers find their seats on their elevator ride. As we approached this part of the ride, fear began to creep in. I got silent as we edged closer and closer, until the moment that we reached the elevator doors. And, y'all...I panicked. I wish I could say I yelled, "Peace out" and smoothly glided out the emergency exit doors without anyone being the wiser. But no, instead I made a humiliating scene, bawled my eyes out, and had the entire elevator ride full of people chanting my name to get on.

Guess what? Even with all of the chanting, cheering, and support, I still didn't get on.

Instead, I made a scene, didn't look back, and left the exit doors to sit outside with my very pregnant mother while we waited for the rest of the crew to exit the ride.

My siblings came out raving about it. They loved it! They had a blast and explained how incredible it was. I was full of regret.

The following trip I made it through the line, conquered my fear, and rode the ride. The second I exited the ride I wanted to do it all over again. My previous fear seemed so silly and miniscule. *What was I even worrying about?*

And right there I learned a valuable lesson.

When you want to do something different or outside of your comfort zone, fear is your mind's automatic defense mechanism. Fear serves as a safety rail to try to keep you from leaving your current state of being and prevent you from making any kind of change.

Fear can, in fact, be helpful in situations in which an actual threat of harm exists—but that's the only place it will ever properly serve you. It's your job to distinguish the two.

Getting out of your comfort zone, facing your fears, and doing something that scares you can actually benefit you tremendously. That's how you learn to live, how to fly the nest, how to make bigger dreams happen.

Take a moment to journal on page 50 of your Toolbook. Can you think of a time as a child when you were scared to do something? What did it feel like? What emotions did you experience?

Now fast forward to your adult life and think: What is something that you have wanted to do, but fear has gotten in the way?

Ask that cute guy out?

Raise your hand in class?

Present at your local MOPs meeting?

There's a reason Fear pops up in those instances. Your mind is literally preventing change. You mind likes safe. Your mind likes comfortable. Your mind likes habit and repetition. Your mind does not like new and different and challenging.

But you have power over your mind. Those things will grow you. Those things will move you. And if you let Fear win, you will forever remain stuck right where you are, thinking about the things that you want to do, giving Fear ultimate control.

When we think about making changes in our lives, sometimes people take a step back because they can't think of a giant dream they've had, or a moment that's going to change their life forever. This does not have to be about dramatic moves that uproot your entire life (unless you're ready for that!). It's about making time for the things your heart keeps leading you to. It's about finding ways to incorporate and work toward fulfilling your passion.

It's about living a life that INSPIRES you.

CHILLS you guys!

So, let's have it...

If money were no obstacle.

If there were no haters to tell you that you can't.

If you could do anything, ANYTHING to make you happy, what would it be? Journal on page 51 of your Toolbook

I love it already.

Now you're going to take the essence of this and incorporate it into your life.

What did you finally admit to yourself that you'd love to do?

Here's what I challenge you to do now.

Give your dream a time stamp.

Here's an example:

VISION: I wanted to write a book. (Hollaaa!)

Now, let's take this a bit deeper and give it a time stamp.

TIME STAMP VISION: I decided two years ago I wanted to create this Toolbook. At the time, I said, "When my daughter is two, I will have the book completed and ready to launch."

Now, maybe it happens sooner. Or, maybe it takes four years instead of three? But guess who's in control of this? Yes, sister, you are.

What goals do you need to accomplish to get to that point?

1. Make a game plan for the subject of your book
2. Write the book
3. Find an editor, publisher, and designer that will support and launch your book
4. Do the dang thing

Do you get the idea here?

Maybe you replace "Writing a book," with opening your own coffee shop, or a nonprofit. Maybe you're not even sure what your big dream is? Maybe you're sitting here thinking, "This is all great for people with a big dream, but that's not me."

If you are stuck at this point, take a break. Take some time to reflect and come back to this. Spend the day soaking in everything around you and see what calls to you. Pay attention to your tiniest thoughts and write them down in the back of your Toolbook in the notes section!

Maybe you end up deciding your vision is just to be a happy, fulfilled family. That's incredible! We can still break it down. As a family, how do you get to this point? Game nights, family dinners, no phones after 7, vacations, budget meetings, etc.?

When it comes time to implement your daily Happy Hour, I would love for you to make some room to pursue this dream—this vision for your life. I want you to take time to focus on your dreams and goals. When you schedule out your weeks and days, I want this to be an important part of your week. Journal your ideas for how to do this on page 53.

In fact, take one hour every day to chase your dream. Instead of watching that extra episode on Netflix, take that hour to do a happy hour task. Instead of sleeping until the kids wake up, wake up an hour earlier and work toward your vision.

Now that we've tackled the entire offensive line, it's time to move to the quarterback (More sports analogies? Who am I?).

Lady, we're going to move on to a vital aspect of your journey. Your physical health.

Step Seven

Step Seven

HEALTH CALL

The Steps so far have all focused on your mental health, serving others, creating happy time, dreaming of your passions, and creating positive thoughts.

Now it's time to chat about your physical health.

Over the next four weeks, you will be moving and shaking!

This is an area that people tend to go head-first into and then burn out quickly because they tired themselves out. The four hours they wanted to spend at the gym after work were too long and eating salads all day every day was exhausting.

So, listen. While I know that it's easy to want to make all the changes at one time, instead, I want you to focus on small steps and consistency over time.

For the next four weeks, I want you to focus on:

1. Moving your body for 20 minutes every single day.
2. Eating at least one fruit or vegetable with every meal.

This doesn't mean you need to train for a marathon (unless that would make you happy!) What this means, is you will be taking time each and every day to move and fuel your body.

This can be dancing, walking, biking, kayaking, rock climbing, following along with a video at home—whatever you can do!

Been dying to sign up for that yoga studio, but been too afraid? NOW IS THE TIME.

Been wanting to join a local hiking club? GO DO IT.

Now if you're someone who hasn't worked out in years, or you feel like you wouldn't even know where to begin, it's okay!

Notice I said, "Movement," not sweating your heart out.

Movement includes *anything* that gets your heart pumping.

You do not have to pay an arm and a leg for a gym membership, unless the movement you'll be committing to at the gym is going to be consistent and make you happy (be HONEST with yourself about this).

If you're starting out from scratch, or working on a budget, walking around your neighborhood is totally free, sister! It doesn't have to cost a lot of money.

Moving can even be setting an alarm on your phone and getting up from your desk to walk around for five minutes, four times a day at work. As long as your body is moving, you're nailing it.

Go for walks during your lunch break.

Get access to workouts from home.

Join that studio you've heard great things about.

Dance it out in your living room to your favorite jams.

You will feel amazing at the end of this!

Again...CHILLS. Journal your ideas for movement on page 61 of your Toolbook.

The next aspect of our Health is one that most people dread.

We are going to talk about what you eat.

Now, I am not going to sit here and tell you to cut out sugar, stop drinking wine, or cut carbs from your life. Instead, I want you to just focus on this one word:

BALANCE.

You can't eat donuts and chips for every single meal and expect to feel energized or Inspired.

Equally, it's not sustainable (or healthy) to swear off any type of food group forever (unless it's due to some type of food allergy).

What you eat has a direct effect on how you feel. If you're

working on your mindset and conquering your fears while filling your body with chips, soda, and skinny vanilla lattes, I can promise that your energy levels will dip really quick. Instead, have the bag of chips with a glass of water. Have your glass of wine while snacking on carrots and hummus instead of binging on the whole sleeve of Oreos.

I don't want this section to be a daunting thing that you dread doing. I want this to be a lifestyle change that fuels your entire life with inspiration. In order to do that, like it or not, you have to show your body some love.

Let's quickly play out a scenario.

It's a Tuesday and your co-worker brings in donuts and coffee to the office.

You can have a donut.

Let me repeat. YOU CAN HAVE A DONUT.

It's what you do after that donut that matters.

After that donut, do you call it a wash, jump down the rabbit hole and ruin the rest of your day with tons of less-than-healthy choices? Maybe eat five more donuts, because, heck you've already had one?

Absolutely not.

After you enjoy every single delicious bite of that donut, you wash it down with some water and go about your day as usual. Having a treat is not the end of the world, so don't treat it like it is (pun totally intended)! There are not "cheat days." There are just regular ol' days with treats included (in moderation).

Two great rules that I've found help me keep it simple are:

1. Include at least one fruit or veggie with every single meal.
2. Drink water all day long. Find a cute water bottle that makes your heart happy and carry it with you everywhere.

One of the hardest things for me when I was first trying to eat healthier was the idea that I couldn't have French fries with every meal (Pregnant Dylan was a different story.) But seriously, I can remember reading through a meal plan, seeing things like, "Replace your side of fries with a side salad or bowl of steamed veggies" and assuming the people who made the plan never had Chick-fil-A before.

Girl, I don't care if you have some fries with that shake. But take a side salad to go and drink your water with it!

We are not dieting. We are not depriving. We are living.

That's it.

I want you to get in the habit of planning out your meals, checking on how you're feeling after certain foods, and beginning to understand what fuels your body and what fails your body.

Once you start planning out your meals and workouts (your movement of choice for the day), you are much more prepared and confident going into every single day without any surprises.

You don't have to spend hours in the kitchen prepping and preparing your meals, unless that's your thing (then more power to you!). But what I do want you to do is have a plan.

Pack your lunch more often. Know what you're going to eat at the restaurant ahead of time, so you're not surprised by the carby options on the menu. And don't be too hard on yourself when Aunt Flo comes to town and all you want are Thin Mints.

It's okay.

Balance, Movement, and Lots of Grace – that's how you really make physical lifestyle changes that last.

In the Weekly Tracker section of your Toolbook, you'll see a place to log your workout and food intake every day. This meal tracking section is not meant to be a place of stress, calorie counting, or deprivation. It is purely there to help you keep track of what you are putting in your body, and then at the end of each day, a place to reflect on how you felt after eating those foods. No guilt, no stress, just things like, "Did this food give me sustained energy, or was I tired 20 minutes later?" "Did this food keep me full, or was I grabbing for pretzels soon after?" Just simply KNOWING how certain foods make you feel can change the game all together and give you access to more intuitive eating habits.

Girl, you're about to change your life.

So now we've talked mindset, power of positivity, serving others, incorporating your happy tasks & scary tasks, movin' and shakin' daily, and balancing your eating habits.

Now, here comes the real nitty gritty stuff, lady...

It's time to put it all into action.

It's time to make a plan in your Toolbook and stick to it!

Implementing Inspiration

IMPLEMENTING INSPIRATION

I want you to pause and give yourself a pat on the back.

Seriously, put this book down and give yourself a big high five, while I currently wrap you in an invisible hug.

Why?

Because I AM SO PROUD OF YOU.

Moving forward and acknowledging deeper powers in our lives is not easy. But You. Are. Doing. It.

You are seven steps closer to living your Inspired life!

I hope that you take other moments outside of this book to really congratulate yourself. Being able to feel pride in things you're doing is a big deal, and is something you should make a point to do.

Sometimes we're so afraid to come off as self-absorbed, that we falter and veer in the opposite direction. Self-loathing, negativity, and overwhelming self-consciousness are NOT how you live Inspired.

Beating yourself down—not okay.

And you're DONE with that kind of life, sister! Those negative emotions do not serve you. If you fall off track...brush your shoulders off and try again. This is your life we're talking about. You have the choice every morning when you wake up to be better, do better, and believe better. So, DO IT!

We already chatted about your mindset and about the role that it plays in your day-to-day life. I want to jump in with one last little exercise with you here.

Let's get hands on with those negative thought processes that so naturally pop up.

Whether it's about a situation, a person, or even about yourself—let's take them and flip the script.

Of course, it's impossible to *only* think positive things, but what if we can combat negative thoughts with our even more powerful positive ones every time?

Need a visual?

I'm reminded of *Star Wars* when I picture negativity and positivity.

Negative thoughts drag you over to "The Dark Side." And who wants to be a Darth Vader? No thanks! (Brutal honesty: This is about as deep as my depth of *Star Wars* knowledge goes. I tried though, right?)

So, instead, what we are going to do is immediately battle negative thoughts with a positive thought.

Picture a green light saber slashing through the red one.

Negativity doesn't stand a chance!

Let me show you some examples.

NEGATIVE THOUGHT: I hate traffic. I'm never going to make it to work on time ...

POSITIVE SPIN: ...but at least I have a job, and I'm safe in my car. Extra time to listen to a podcast or my favorite songs!

NEGATIVE THOUGHT: Ugh this skirt is way too small; I'm never going to fit in a size two ever again

POSITIVE SPIN: ...but this body supported an entire life form. How cool is it that these hips and this belly held a child?! And look how stinkin' strong my arms look—hello!

NEGATIVE THOUGHT: My co-worker is the absolute worst. I can't believe she is so rude! And to make me do all of this work on my own...

POSITIVE SPIN: ...but I am so capable of doing anything. She must be in a super negative place to try to bring me down like that, and it's not going to work. Maybe I'll invite her to join me for a yoga class soon.

At first, it will take reminding to create these positive spins. And it may feel a little silly, or even awkward and forced. But I promise that once you get the hang of it, it will make all the difference in how you combat your mind's negativity.

Worried you'll have a hard time coming up with positive spins?

On page 68 of your Toolbook, write a list of things you are thankful for—things that bring you joy in your everyday, things you love about yourself, things you love about others. These will serve as tools that you can use when those negative thoughts arise.

Now you can immediately begin using this tool to combat negative thoughts by referring to it every time you have a negative thought about a situation, yourself, or someone else. Every time you have a negative thought, replace it with a positive thought from your thankful list.

Maybe as you're making these lists, negativity is creeping in. Bring in some girlfriends and family members and get their help coming up with some positivity brainstorming!

Need a reminder to focus on these things each day?

Try setting the background on your phone to a picture that makes you happy and reminds you to combat negativity.

Wear a hair tie around your wrist that you can look down at and remember three positive things.

Heck, tattoo that positivity on yourself and focus on reminding yourself for life.

Because, sister, YOU ARE AMAZING!

You are powerful.

You are a warrior princess who is about to take your life to the next level.

You feel that power??

This is YOU. This is who YOU WERE MADE TO BE.

Ready to begin your Inspired lifestyle?

Your next steps are simple. It's time to take it to the Toolbook.

What you will be doing now is taking everything you just learned and implementing it daily.

And I'm going to be completely honest with you—it's your turn to decide if you are ready for it. It's your turn to actually go after those things, to complete the next four weeks of your Toolbook, to decide that you want this Inspired life.

The word discipline so often gets a negative connotation. We think of spankings and time-out, we think of getting in trouble, or even some form of terrible strictness. But, sister, I want you to focus on the self-loving discipline it will take for you to complete these next four weeks.

I've been here, walking you through these first sections, and I'll be here with you even then, but I need you to show up with me. Even when it's hard, even when you're tired, even when you're afraid, even when all you want is to curl up in a ball and binge watch *Friends* on Netflix—I want you to SHOW UP for your life.

Your mind will naturally give you a second "Is this a good idea?" thought before taking a step forward and taking action. I challenge you, in those moments when you want to give up on yourself, when you want to forget to write in your Toolbook for a day, to just show BACK UP.
This is your life we're talking about. You owe it to yourself to have the discipline. Like a BFF refusing to let her bestie take

back that cheating ex, YOU have to decide that you're going to do this day in and day out. And, girlfriend, if you can do that, your life is going to be AMAZING.

For the next 30 days, your job is to just do it! I'm not asking you to try to do it or hope that your life is going to change.

I challenge you to take action and intentionally make the necessary changes.

You will spend every single day focusing on these seven steps:

1. You WILL control the controllable and let go of the rest.
2. You WILL master your mindset.
3. You WILL chase your dreams.
4. You WILL serve others.
5. You WILL do something for yourself daily.
6. You WILL conquer your fears.
7. You WILL take control of your health and wellness.

Reading through that, how do you feel?

You should feel ON FIRE, SIS!

Now, one final challenge. I want you to sign your name on the line below to signify your commit to making the changes necessary, day in and day out.

I promise you are going to live in the most Inspired way possible, girlfriend. And I can't wait to watch!

Don't forget to tag me, share your testimonials, share your stories, and join #TheInspiredSisterhood online!

I am committed to living my Inspired life, starting right now.

X _____

See you on the other side, sister!

XO,
Dylan